DIABETES COOKBOOK
FOR BLACK PEOPLE

Discover Flavorful Recipes for
Managing Diabetes in the
Black Community

Diane J. Hays

DISCLAIMER

The information in this book is for educational purposes only and should not be considered medical advice. Consult a healthcare professional before making any dietary or lifestyle changes. The author is not liable for any consequences resulting from the use of this book.

TABLE OF CONTENTS

DIABETES COOKBOOK
FOR BLACK PEOPLE

INTRODUCTION

Welcome to the culinary world of "Diabetes Cookbook for Black People." In the diverse landscape of Black cuisine, food is not only nourishment but also a celebration of heritage, community, and resilience. However, managing diabetes within this cultural context can present unique challenges, as traditional flavors and culinary practices intersect with the need for balanced nutrition and blood sugar management.

But fear not, for this cookbook is here to guide you on a flavorful and empowering journey towards health and wellness. With a focus on the rich culinary traditions of the Black community, "Diabetes Cookbook for Black People" offers a curated collection of delicious recipes designed specifically for individuals managing diabetes.

Within these pages, you'll discover an abundance of mouthwatering dishes that marry the bold flavors of our cultural heritage with the nutritional principles necessary for diabetes management. From soulful classics to contemporary favorites, each recipe is a testament to the power of food to nourish both body and soul.

Whether you're seeking to stabilize blood sugar levels, improve overall health, or simply indulge in the flavors of home in a mindful way, "Diabetes Cookbook for Black People" is your trusted companion. Get ready to explore the vibrant world of Black cuisine while reclaiming control of your health and vitality. Let's embark on this delicious journey together, one recipe at a time.

CHAPTER ONE

Breakfast

Introduction:

Welcome to the Breakfast chapter of "Diabetes Cookbook for Black People." A nourishing start to the day sets the tone for healthy eating and blood sugar management. In this chapter, we've curated six flavorful breakfast recipes that celebrate the rich culinary heritage of the Black community while supporting your journey to optimal health and wellness.

1. Sweet Potato Breakfast Hash

- Cook Time: 20 minutes

- Servings: 4

- Ingredients:

  - Sweet potatoes of two medium sizes should be peeled and diced

  - 1 bell pepper, diced

  - 1 onion, diced

  - 2 cloves garlic, minced

- 4 links turkey sausage, sliced

- 1 tablespoon olive oil

- Salt and pepper to taste

- Instructions:

1. Heat olive oil in a skillet on average heat. Add diced sweet potatoes and cook until slightly softened, about 5 minutes.

2. Add diced bell pepper, onion, garlic, and turkey sausage to the skillet. Cook until vegetables are tender and sausage is browned, about 10 minutes.

3. Apply with salt and pepper to taste and serve.

- Nutritional Info:

- Calories: 250

- Carbohydrates: 30g

- Protein: 15g

- Fat: 8g

- Fiber: 5g

2. Jamaican Ackee and Saltfish

- Cook Time: 20 minutes

- Servings: 4

- Ingredients:

  - 1 can ackee, drained

  - 1 cup salted cod fish, soaked and shredded

  - 1 onion, chopped

  - 1 bell pepper, chopped

  - 2 tomatoes, chopped

  - 2 cloves garlic, minced

  - 1 scotch bonnet pepper, chopped (optional)

  - 2 tablespoons olive oil

- Instructions:

1. Heat olive oil on average heat in a skillet. Chop onion, bell pepper, tomatoes, and garlic and add them togethe and. cook until softened, about five minutes.

2. Add shredded salted cod fish and cook for another 5 minutes.

3. Gently fold in drained ackee and scotch bonnet pepper (if using). Cook for more five

minutes while you continue to stir it to combine. Serve hot.

- Nutritional Info:

  - Calories: 280

  - Carbohydrates: 15g

  - Protein: 20g

  - Fat: 12g

  - Fiber: 3g

3. Southern Style Grits with Shrimp

- Cook Time: 20 minutes

- Servings: 4

- Ingredients:

  - 1 cup stone-ground grits

  - 2 cups water

  - 2 cups low-sodium chicken broth

  - 1 cup shredded cheddar cheese

    - Provide one pound of medium shrimp, peeled and deveined

  - 2 tablespoons butter

  - Salt and pepper to taste

- Instructions:

1. In a saucepan, bring water and chicken broth to a boil. Slowly whisk in grits, reduce heat to low, and simmer until thickened, about 15 minutes.

2. Stir in shredded cheddar cheese and butter until melted and creamy. Apply salt and pepper to season and taste.

3. In a separate skillet, cook shrimp until pink and opaque, about 3-4 minutes per side.

4. Serve shrimp over a bed of creamy grits. Enjoy hot.

- Nutritional Info:

  - Calories: 350

  - Carbohydrates: 25g

  - Protein: 25g

  - Fat: 15g

  - Fiber: 2g

4. Plantain and Black Bean Breakfast Bowl

- Cook Time: 15 minutes

- Servings: 2

- Ingredients:

- 2 ripe plantains, sliced

- 1 can black beans, drained and rinsed

- 1 avocado, sliced

- 2 eggs

- 2 tablespoons olive oil

- Salt and pepper to taste

- Instructions:

1. On average heat, heat olive oil in a skillet. Add sliced plantains and cook until golden brown on both sides, about 5 minutes per side. Remove from skillet and set aside.

2. In the same skillet, add black beans and heat until warmed through, about 3-4 minutes.

3. Meanwhile, fry eggs to desired doneness in a separate skillet.

4. Assemble breakfast bowls with plantains, black beans, avocado slices, and fried eggs. Season with salt and pepper to taste. Serve hot.

- Nutritional Info:

- Calories: 400

- Carbohydrates: 40g

- Protein: 15g

- Fat: 20g

- Fiber: 10g

5. Spinach and Feta Egg Muffins

- Cook Time: 20 minutes

- Servings: 6

- Ingredients:

  - 6 eggs

  - 1 cup fresh spinach, chopped

  - 1/2 cup crumbled feta cheese

  - 1/4 cup diced tomatoes

  - 2 tablespoons chopped fresh parsley

  - Salt and pepper to taste

- Instructions:

  1. Preheat oven to 350°F (175°C). Grease a muffin tin with cooking spray.

  2. In a bowl, whisk together eggs, chopped spinach, crumbled feta cheese, diced tomatoes, chopped fresh parsley , salt, and pepper.

3. Pour egg mixture into prepared muffin tin, filling each cup about 3/4 full.

4. Bake in the preheated oven for 15-20 minutes, or until eggs are set and muffins are golden brown.

5. Allow muffins to cool slightly before removing from the tin. Serve warm.

- Nutritional Info:

  - Calories: 120

  - Carbohydrates: 2g

  - Protein: 8g

  - Fat: 9g

  - Fiber: 1g

6. Caribbean Coconut Porridge

- Cook Time: 20 minutes

- Servings: 4

- Ingredients:

  - 1 cup cornmeal

  - 4 cups coconut milk

  - Provide quarter cup of brown sugar

  - 1 teaspoon vanilla extract

- 1/2 teaspoon ground cinnamon

- Pinch of salt

1. In a saucepan, whisk together cornmeal and coconut milk until smooth.

2. Place saucepan over medium heat and bring mixture to a simmer, stirring constantly.

3. Reduce heat to low and continue to cook, stirring frequently, until porridge thickens, about 15-20 minutes.

4. Stir in brown sugar or maple syrup, vanilla extract, ground cinnamon, and a pinch of salt. Cook for an additional 2-3 minutes.

5. Serve warm, garnished with additional cinnamon if desired.

- Nutritional Info:

- Calories: 200

- Carbohydrates: 25g

- Protein: 2g

- Fat: 10g

- Fiber: 2g

DIABETES COOKBOOK
FOR BLACK PEOPLE

Chapter Two

CHAPTER TWO

<u>Soups and Stews</u>

Introduction:

Welcome to the Soups and Stews chapter of "Diabetes Cookbook for Black People." A warm bowl of soup or stew is not just a meal; it's a comforting embrace, a taste of home, and a celebration of culinary heritage. In this chapter, we've curated six hearty recipes that pay homage to the diverse flavors and traditions of the Black community while supporting your health and well-being.

1. Creole Chicken and Okra Gumbo

- Cook Time: 1 hour

- Servings: 6

- Ingredients:

  - 1 pound boneless, skinless chicken thighs, diced

  - 1 onion, chopped

  - 1 bell pepper, chopped

- 2 stalks celery, chopped

- 2 cloves garlic, minced

- 1 cup sliced okra

- 1 can diced tomatoes

- 4 cups low-sodium chicken broth

- 1 teaspoon dried thyme

- 1 teaspoon dried oregano

- 1/2 teaspoon paprika

- Salt and pepper to taste

- Instructions:

1. Heat olive oil on average heat in a big pot. Add diced chicken thighs and cook until browned, about 5 minutes.

2. Add chopped onion, bell pepper, celery, and garlic to the pot. Cook until vegetables are softened, about 5 minutes.

3. Stir in sliced okra, diced tomatoes, chicken broth, dried thyme, dried oregano, paprika, salt, and pepper. Bring to a boil, then reduce heat and simmer for 30-40 minutes.

4. Serve hot, garnished with chopped fresh parsley if desired.

- Nutritional Info:

  - Calories: 250

  - Carbohydrates: 15g

  - Protein: 20g

  - Fat: 8g

  - Fiber: 5g

2. Caribbean Red Pea Soup

- Cook Time: 1 hour 30 minutes
- Servings: 6
- Ingredients:

   - One cup of dried red kidney beans should be soaked through the night and drained

  - 1 onion, chopped

  - 2 carrots, chopped

  - 2 stalks celery, chopped

  - 2 cloves garlic, minced

  - 1 can coconut milk

  - 4 cups vegetable broth

  - 1 teaspoon ground allspice

  - 1/2 teaspoon dried thyme

  - 1 bay leaf

- Salt and pepper to taste

- Instructions:

1. In a large pot, combine soaked red kidney beans, chopped onion, carrots, celery, garlic, coconut milk, vegetable broth, ground allspice, dried thyme, bay leaf, salt, and pepper.

2. Bring to a boil, then reduce heat and simmer for 1 hour to 1 hour 30 minutes, or until beans are tender.

3. Remove bay leaf and discard. Use an immersion blender to blend soup to desired consistency.

4. Serve hot, garnished with chopped fresh parsley if desired.

- Nutritional Info:

- Calories: 300

- Carbohydrates: 25g

- Protein: 10g

- Fat: 15g

- Fiber: 8g

3. West African Peanut Stew

- Cook Time: 45 minutes

- Servings: 6

- Ingredients:

  - 1 tablespoon olive oil

  - 1 onion, chopped

  - 2 carrots, chopped

  - 2 sweet potatoes, peeled and diced

  - 2 cloves garlic, minced

  - 1 teaspoon grated ginger

  - 1/2 teaspoon ground cumin

  - 1/2 teaspoon ground coriander

  - 1/4 teaspoon cayenne pepper

  - 1/2 cup smooth peanut butter

  - 4 cups vegetable broth

  - 1 can diced tomatoes

  - 2 cups chopped collard greens

  - Salt and pepper to taste

- Instructions:

  1. Heat olive oil on heat in a big pot. Add
     chopped onion, carrots, and sweet

potatoes. Cook until vegetables are softened, about 5 minutes.

2. Add minced garlic, grated ginger, ground cumin, ground coriander, and cayenne pepper to the pot. Cook for another 2 minutes.

3. Stir in smooth peanut butter until combined, then add vegetable broth and diced tomatoes. Bring to a simmer and cook for 20-25 minutes.

4. Add chopped collard greens to the pot and cook for an additional 5 minutes, or until greens are tender.

5. Serve hot, garnished with chopped roasted peanuts if desired.

- Nutritional Info:

- Calories: 350

- Carbohydrates: 30g

- Protein: 15g

- Fat: 20g

- Fiber: 8g

4. Caribbean Pumpkin Soup

- Cook Time: 45 minutes

- Servings: 6

- Ingredients:

  - 1 tablespoon olive oil

  - 1 onion, chopped

  - 2 cloves garlic, minced

  - 1 teaspoon grated ginger

  - 1 teaspoon ground allspice

  - 1/2 teaspoon ground cinnamon

  - 1/4 teaspoon ground nutmeg

  - 4 cups vegetable broth

  - 4 cups diced pumpkin or butternut squash

  - 1 can coconut milk

  - One tablespoon of brown sugar

  - Salt and pepper to taste

- Instructions:

  1. Heat olive oil on average heat in a big pot, chop onion and cook for about five to six minutes to make it soft.

2. Add minced garlic, grated ginger, ground allspice, ground cinnamon, and ground nutmeg to the pot. Cook for another 2 minutes.

3. Stir in vegetable broth, diced pumpkin or butternut squash, coconut milk, and brown sugar or maple syrup. Boil and then decrease heat and simmer for twenty five to thirty minutes until it's soft.

4. Use an immersion blender to blend soup until smooth. Apply salt and pepper to season and taste.

5. Serve hot, garnished with a drizzle of coconut milk and a sprinkle of ground cinnamon if desired.

- Nutritional Info:

- Calories: 200

- Carbohydrates: 25g

- Protein: 3g

- Fat: 10g

- Fiber: 5g

5. Southern Corn and Crab Chowder

- Cook Time: 40 minutes

- Servings: 6

- Ingredients:

  - 1 tablespoon olive oil

  - 1 onion, chopped

  - 2 stalks celery, chopped

  - 1 bell pepper, chopped

  - 2 cloves garlic, minced

  - 4 cups low-sodium chicken broth

  - 2 cups frozen corn kernels

  - One can of lump crab meat should be drained

  - 1 cup heavy cream

  - 1 teaspoon Old Bay seasoning

  - Salt and pepper to taste

- Instructions:

  1. Heat olive oil on average heat in a big pot. Add chopped onion, celery, bell pepper, and garlic. Cook until vegetables are softened, about 5 minutes.

2. Stir in chicken broth, frozen corn kernels, lump crab meat, heavy cream, and Old Bay seasoning. Bring to a simmer and cook for 20-25 minutes.

3. Apply salt and pepper to to season and taste.

4. Serve hot, garnished with chopped fresh parsley if desired.

- Nutritional Info:

  - Calories: 300

  - Carbohydrates: 20g

  - Protein: 15g

  - Fat: 15g

  - Fiber: 3g

6. Jamaican Beef Stew

- Cook Time: 1 hour 30 minutes

- Servings: 6

- Ingredients:

  - 1 tablespoon olive oil

  - Two pounds of beef stew meat and cut them into cubes

  - 1 onion, chopped

- 2 carrots, chopped

- 2 stalks celery, chopped

- 2 cloves garlic, minced

- 2 cups beef broth

- 1 can diced tomatoes

- 1 tablespoon Worcestershire sauce

- 1 teaspoon dried thyme

- 1 teaspoon paprika

- Salt and pepper to taste

- Instructions:

1. Heat olive oil in a big pot. Add beef stew meat and cook until browned on all sides, about 5-7 minutes.

2. Add chopped onion, carrots, celery, and garlic to the pot. Cook until vegetables are softened, about 5 minutes.

3. Stir in beef broth, diced tomatoes, Worcestershire sauce, dried thyme, paprika, salt, and pepper. Bring to a boil, then reduce heat and simmer for 1 hour to 1 hour 30 minutes, or until beef is tender.

4. Serve hot, garnished with chopped fresh parsley if desired.

- Nutritional Info:

- Calories: 350

- Carbohydrates: 10g

- Protein: 25g

- Fat: 20g

- Fiber: 2g

CHAPTER THREE

<u>Main Dishes</u>

Introduction:

Welcome to the Main Dish chapter of "Diabetes Cookbook for Black People." In this chapter, we celebrate the heart of the meal—the main course. From savory and satisfying meat dishes to flavorful vegetarian options, these recipes are sure to delight your taste buds while supporting your journey to managing diabetes with delicious and nutritious meals.

1. Jamaican Jerk Chicken

- Cook Time: 45 minutes

- Servings: 4

- Ingredients:

  - 4 bone-in, skin-on chicken thighs

  - 1/4 cup Jamaican jerk seasoning

  - 2 tablespoons olive oil

  - 1 lime, juiced

  - Salt to taste

1. Preheat oven to 375°F (190°C).

2. In a bowl, combine Jamaican jerk seasoning, olive oil, lime juice, and salt.

3. Apply mixture of the seasoning mixture over the chicken thighs.

4. On a baking sheet lined with parchment paper place chicken thighs

5. Bake in the preheated oven for 35-40 minutes, or until chicken is cooked through and skin is crispy.

6. Garnished with fresh cilantro if wishes and serve.

- Nutritional Info:

  - Calories: 300
  - Carbohydrates: 0g
  - Protein: 25g
  - Fat: 20g
  - Fiber: 0g

2. Soulful Collard Greens

- Cook Time: 1 hour

- Ingredients:

  - 2 bunches collard greens, stems removed and leaves chopped
  - 4 slices smoked turkey bacon, chopped
  - 1 onion, chopped
  - 2 cloves garlic, minced
  - 2 cups low-sodium chicken broth
  - 1 tablespoon apple cider vinegar
  - Salt and pepper to taste

- Instructions:

1. In a large pot, cook chopped turkey bacon over medium heat until crispy.

2. Chop onion and minced garlic and add them to the pot. Cook until softened, about 5 minutes.

3. Stir in chopped collard greens, chicken broth, apple cider vinegar, salt, and pepper.

4. Boil decrease the heat a bit lower. Cover and simmer for 45-60 minutes, or until collard greens are tender.

5. Serve hot, with a splash of hot sauce if desired.

- Nutritional Info:

- Calories: 100

- Carbohydrates: 10g

- Protein: 5g

- Fat: 5g

- Fiber: 5g

3. Cajun Blackened Catfish

- Cook Time: 20 minutes

- Servings: 4

- Ingredients:

- 4 catfish fillets

- 2 tablespoons Cajun seasoning

- 2 tablespoons olive oil

- 1 lemon, cut into wedges

- Salt to taste

- Instructions:

1. Rub Cajun seasoning all over the catfish fillets, ensuring they are evenly coated.

2. Heat olive oil in a skillet over medium-high heat.

3. Add catfish fillets to the skillet and cook for 4-5 minutes per side, or until fish flakes easily with a fork and is blackened.

4. Squeeze fresh lemon juice over the cooked catfish fillets and sprinkle with salt.

5. Serve hot, with additional lemon wedges on the side.

- Nutritional Info:

  - Calories: 200

  - Carbohydrates: 0g

  - Protein: 20g

  - Fat: 10g

  - Fiber: 0g

4. Vegan Jollof Rice

- Cook Time: 45 minutes

- Servings: 6

- Ingredients:

  - 2 cups long-grain white rice

  - 1 onion, chopped

- 2 cloves garlic, minced

- 1 bell pepper, chopped

- 1 can diced tomatoes

- 2 cups vegetable broth

- 1 teaspoon paprika

- 1/2 teaspoon dried thyme

- 1/2 teaspoon curry powder

- Salt and pepper to taste

- Instructions:

1. Heat olive oil on average heat in a big pot. Add chopped onion, minced garlic, and chopped bell pepper. Cook until softened, about 5 minutes.

2. Stir in diced tomatoes, vegetable broth, paprika, dried thyme, curry powder, salt, and pepper.

3. Boil and then decrease the heat a bit lower. Put the rice in the pot and stir to mix them gently.

4. Cover and simmer for 20-25 minutes, or until rice is cooked and liquid is absorbed.

5. Serve hot, garnished with chopped fresh parsley if desired.

- Nutritional Info:

  - Calories: 250

  - Carbohydrates: 50g

  - Protein: 5g

  - Fat: 2g

  - Fiber: 3g

5. Southern Baked Catfish

- Cook Time: 25 minutes

- Servings: 4

- Ingredients:

  - 4 catfish fillets

  - 1/2 cup cornmeal

  - 1 teaspoon paprika

  - 1/2 teaspoon garlic powder

  - 1/2 teaspoon onion powder

  - 1/4 teaspoon cayenne pepper

  - 2 tablespoons olive oil

  - Lemon wedges for serving

  - Salt and pepper to taste

1. Preheat oven to 400°F (200°C). Line a baking sheet with parchment paper.

2. Combine and mix cornmeal, paprika, garlic powder, onion powder, cayenne pepper, salt, and pepper in a shallow dish.

3. Pat catfish fillets dry with paper towels. Dip each fillet into the cornmeal mixture, coating both sides evenly.

4. Place coated catfish fillets on the prepared baking sheet. Drizzle olive oil over the fillets.

5. Bake in the preheated oven for 20-25 minutes, or until fish is cooked through and flakes easily with a fork.

6. Serve hot, with lemon wedges on the side.

- Calories: 300

- Carbohydrates: 15g

- Protein: 20g

- Fat: 15g

- Fiber: 1g

6. Vegan Stuffed Bell Peppers

- Cook Time: 45 minutes

- Servings: 6

- Ingredients:

  - 6 bell peppers, tops removed and seeds removed

  - 1 cup quinoa, cooked

  - 1 can black beans, drained and rinsed

  - - 1 cup corn kernels

  - 1 onion, chopped

  - 2 cloves garlic, minced

  - 1 can diced tomatoes

  - 1 teaspoon ground cumin

  - 1 teaspoon chili powder

  - Salt and pepper to taste

  - 1/2 cup shredded vegan cheese (optional)

- Instructions:

  1. Preheat oven to 375°F (190°C).

  2. Heat olive oil on average heat in a big skillet. Add chopped onion and minced garlic. Cook until softened, about 5 minutes.

3. Add cooked quinoa, black beans, corn kernels, diced tomatoes, ground cumin, chili powder, salt, and pepper to the skillet. Cook for an additional 5 minutes, until heated through.

4. Put quinoa with bell pepper each and black bean mixture.

5. Place stuffed bell peppers in a baking dish. Sprinkle shredded vegan cheese over them.

6. Bake in the preheated oven for 25-30 minutes, until bell peppers are tender.

7. Serve hot, garnished with chopped fresh cilantro if desired.

- Nutritional Info:

  - Calories: 200

  - Carbohydrates: 35g

  - Protein: 8g

  - Fat: 3g

  - Fiber: 8g

CHAPTER FOUR

Sides and Salads

Introduction:

Welcome to the Sides and Salads chapter of "Diabetes Cookbook for Black People." A well-rounded meal isn't complete without delicious side dishes and refreshing salads to complement the main course. In this chapter, we've curated a collection of vibrant salads and flavorful sides that celebrate the bounty of fresh ingredients and diverse flavors. These recipes are perfect for adding color, texture, and nutrition to your plate while managing your diabetes with confidence and enjoyment.

1. Southern Collard Greens Salad

- Prep Time:15 minutes
- Servings: 4
- Ingredients:

  - 1 bunch collard greens, stems removed and leaves thinly sliced

- 1/4 cup apple cider vinegar

- 2 tablespoons olive oil

- 1 teaspoon Dijon mustard

- One tablespoon of honey

- 1/4 cup chopped pecans, toasted

- Salt and pepper to taste

- Instructions:

1. In a large bowl, whisk together apple cider vinegar, olive oil, Dijon mustard, honey or maple syrup, salt, and pepper to make the dressing.

2. Add thinly sliced collard greens to the bowl and toss to coat with the dressing.

3. Let the salad sit for at least 10 minutes to allow the flavors to meld.

4. Sprinkle toasted pecans over the salad just before serving.

- Nutritional Info:

- Calories: 150

- Carbohydrates: 10g

- Protein: 3g

- Fat: 12g

- Fiber: 4g

2. Creole Roasted Sweet Potatoes

- Prep Time: 10 minutes

- Cook Time: 30 minutes

- Servings: 4

- Ingredients:

  - 2 large sweet potatoes, peeled and cubed

  - 2 tablespoons olive oil

  - 1 teaspoon Creole seasoning

  - 1/2 teaspoon smoked paprika

  - 1/4 teaspoon cayenne pepper

  - Salt and pepper to taste

- Instructions:

  1. Preheat oven to 400°F (200°C) and line a baking sheet with parchment paper.

  2. In a large bowl, toss cubed sweet potatoes with olive oil, Creole seasoning, smoked paprika, cayenne pepper, salt, and pepper until evenly coated.

  3. Spread the seasoned sweet potatoes in a single layer on the prepared baking sheet.

4. Roast in the preheated oven for 25-30 minutes, or until sweet potatoes are tender and caramelized, stirring halfway through.

5. Serve hot as a flavorful side dish.

- Nutritional Info:

  - Calories: 180

  - Carbohydrates: 25g

  - Protein: 2g

  - Fat: 8g

  - Fiber: 4g

3. Caribbean Mango and Avocado Salad

- Prep Time: 15 minutes

- Servings: 4

- Ingredients:

  - Two ripe mangoes should be peeled, pitted, and diced

  - Two ripe avocados should be peeled, pitted, and diced

  - 1/4 cup red onion, finely chopped

  - 1/4 cup fresh cilantro, chopped

  - 1 lime, juiced

- 1 tablespoon olive oil

- Salt and pepper to taste

- Instructions:

1. In a large bowl, combine diced mangoes, diced avocados, chopped red onion, and chopped fresh cilantro.

2. Drizzle lime juice and olive oil over the salad, and season with salt and pepper to taste.

3. Gently toss until all ingredients are evenly coated with the dressing.

4. Serve chilled as a refreshing salad or side dish.

- Nutritional Info:

- Calories: 200

- Carbohydrates: 20g

- Protein: 2g

- Fat: 14g

- Fiber: 7g

4. Southern Style Green Beans

- Prep Time: 10 minutes

- Cook Time: 15 minutes

- Servings: 4

- Ingredients:

  - 1 pound fresh green beans, trimmed

  - 2 slices turkey bacon, chopped

  - 1/4 cup onion, finely chopped

  - 1 clove garlic, minced

  - 1 tablespoon apple cider vinegar

  - 1 tablespoon olive oil

  - Salt and pepper to taste

- Instructions:

  1. In a large skillet, cook chopped turkey bacon over medium heat until crispy.

  2. Chop onion and minced garlic and add them to the skillet. Cook until softened, about 3-4 minutes.

  3. Add trimmed green beans to the skillet and cook until tender-crisp, about 5-7 minutes.

  4. Drizzle apple cider vinegar and olive oil over the green beans, and season with salt and pepper to taste.

5. Toss to coat evenly and cook for an additional 2-3 minutes.

6. Serve hot as a classic Southern side dish.

- Nutritional Info:

  - Calories: 120

  - Carbohydrates: 12g

  - Protein: 4g

  - Fat: 7g

  - Fiber: 5g

5. Cajun Coleslaw

- Prep Time: 10 minutes

- Servings: 4

- Ingredients:

  - Four cups of shredded cabbage

  -- 1/2 cup shredded carrots

  - 1/4 cup chopped green onions

  - 1/4 cup mayonnaise

  - 2 tablespoons apple cider vinegar

  - 1 tablespoon Dijon mustard

  - 1 teaspoon Cajun seasoning

  - Salt and pepper to taste

1. In a large bowl, combine shredded cabbage, shredded carrots, and chopped green onions.

2. In a separate small bowl, whisk together mayonnaise, apple cider vinegar, Dijon mustard, Cajun seasoning, salt, and pepper to make the dressing.

3. Pour the dressing over the cabbage mixture and toss until evenly coated.

4. Put in a refrigerator for at least thirty minutes before serving for the flavors to meld.

5. Serve chilled as a zesty and flavorful side dish.

- Nutritional Info:

  - Calories: 150

  - Carbohydrates: 8g

  - Protein: 1g

  - Fat: 12g

  - Fiber: 3g

6. Jamaican Rice and Peas

- Prep Time: 10 minutes

- Cook Time: 45 minutes

- Servings: 4

- Ingredients:

  - 1 cup long-grain white rice

  - One can of red kidney beans should be drained and rinsed

  - 1 cup coconut milk

  - 1 cup water

  - 2 cloves garlic, minced

  - 1 teaspoon dried thyme

  - 1 teaspoon allspice

  - Salt and pepper to taste

- Instructions:

  1. In a large pot, combine rice, red kidney beans, coconut milk, water, minced garlic, dried thyme, allspice, salt, and pepper.

  2. On high heat, boil the mixture.

  3. Once boiling, reduce the heat to low, cover, and simmer for 30-35 minutes, or until the rice is cooked and the liquid is absorbed.

4. Take the pot away from the heat and let it covered for about five minutes.

5. Fluff the rice with a fork before serving.

- Nutritional Info:

  - Calories: 250

  - Carbohydrates: 45g

  - Protein: 7g

  - Fat: 5g

  - Fiber: 6g

CHAPTER FIVE

Desserts

Introduction:

Indulge your sweet tooth guilt-free with the delightful desserts in this chapter of "Diabetes Cookbook for Black People." From classic favorites with a healthy twist to inventive treats bursting with flavor, these desserts are sure to satisfy your cravings while helping you manage your diabetes. Whether you're craving something creamy, fruity, or chocolaty, there's a dessert here for every occasion and every palate. So go ahead, treat yourself to something sweet and delicious without worrying about your blood sugar levels.

1. Banana Pudding Parfait

- Prep Time: 15 minutes

- Chill Time: 2 hours

- Servings: 4

- Ingredients:

- 2 ripe bananas, mashed

- 1 cup low-fat vanilla Greek yogurt

- 1/2 cup crushed vanilla wafer cookies

- 1/4 cup chopped pecans

- 1/4 cup unsweetened shredded coconut

- Instructions:

1. In a small bowl, mix together mashed bananas and low-fat vanilla Greek yogurt until well combined.

2. In serving glasses or bowls, layer the banana-yogurt mixture with crushed vanilla wafer cookies, chopped pecans, and shredded coconut.

3. Repeat the layers until the glasses or bowls are filled, ending with a sprinkle of crushed vanilla wafer cookies on top.

4. Cover and refrigerate for at least 2 hours, or until chilled and set.

5. Serve cold as a delicious and satisfying dessert.

- Nutritional Info:

- Calories: 200

- Carbohydrates: 25g

- Protein: 8g

- Fat: 8g

- Fiber: 3g

2. Berry Almond Crisp

- Prep Time: 15 minutes

- Bake Time: 35 minutes

- Servings: 6

- Ingredients:

   - Four cups of mixed berries like strawberries, blueberries and or raspberries

   - 1 tablespoon lemon juice

   - 1/4 cup almond flour

   - 1/4 cup rolled oats

   - 1/4 cup sliced almonds

   - 2 tablespoons maple syrup

   - 1 tablespoon coconut oil, melted

   - 1/2 teaspoon ground cinnamon

- Instructions:

   1. Preheat oven to 350°F (175°C). Grease a baking dish with coconut oil.

2. In a large bowl, toss mixed berries with lemon juice until evenly coated. Prepare a baking dish and place the berries onto it.

3. In the same bowl, combine almond flour, rolled oats, sliced almonds, maple syrup, melted coconut oil, and ground cinnamon. Mix until crumbly.

4. Sprinkle the almond-oat mixture evenly over the berries in the baking dish.

5. Bake in the preheated oven for 30-35 minutes, or until the berries are bubbling and the topping is golden brown.

6. Remove from the oven and let cool slightly before serving.

- Nutritional Info:

- Calories: 180

- Carbohydrates: 25g

- Protein: 5g

- Fat: 8g

- Fiber: 6g

3. Chocolate Avocado Mousse

- Prep Time: 10 minutes

- Chill Time: 1 hour

- Servings: 4

- Ingredients:

  - 2 ripe avocados, peeled and pitted

  - 1/4 cup unsweetened cocoa powder

  - 1/4 cup maple syrup

  - 2 tablespoons almond milk

  - 1 teaspoon vanilla extract

- Instructions:

1. In a food processor or blender, combine peeled and pitted avocados, unsweetened cocoa powder, maple syrup, almond milk, and vanilla extract.

2. Blend until smooth and creamy, scraping down the sides as needed.

3. Divide the chocolate avocado mousse into serving glasses or bowls.

4. Cover and refrigerate for at least 1 hour, or until chilled and set.

5. Serve cold as a rich and indulgent dessert.

- Nutritional Info:

  - Calories: 200

  - Carbohydrates: 15g

  - Protein: 3g

  - Fat: 15g

  - Fiber: 7g

4. Pineapple Coconut Sorbet

- Prep Time: 10 minutes

- Chill Time: 4 hours

- Servings: 6

- Ingredients:

  - 4 cups frozen pineapple chunks

  - 1/2 cup canned coconut milk

  - 2 tablespoons maple syrup

  - 1 tablespoon lime juice

- Instructions:

1. In a blender, combine frozen pineapple chunks, canned coconut milk, maple syrup, and lime juice.

2. Blend until smooth and creamy, scraping down the sides as needed.

3. Transfer the mixture to a shallow dish and spread it out evenly.

4. Cover and freeze for at least 4 hours, or until firm.

5. Allow the sorbet to sit under room temperature for some minutes to soften it a bit before serving.

6. Serve scoops of pineapple coconut sorbet in bowls or cones.

- Nutritional Info:

  - Calories: 120

  - Carbohydrates: 20g

  - Protein: 1g

  - Fat: 5g

  - Fiber: 3g

5. Peach Cobbler

- Prep Time: 15 minutes

- Bake Time: 40 minutes

- Servings: 6

- Ingredients:

  - 4 cups sliced peaches (fresh or frozen)

- 1 tablespoon lemon juice

- Quarter cup of maple syrup

- 1 teaspoon vanilla extract

- 1 cup almond flour

- 1/4 cup rolled oats

- 1/4 cup sliced almonds

- 2 tablespoons coconut oil, melted

- 1/2 teaspoon ground cinnamon

- Instructions:

1. Preheat oven to 350°F (175°C). Grease a baking dish with coconut oil.

2. In a large bowl, toss sliced peaches with lemon juice, maple syrup, and vanilla extract until evenly coated. Transfer the peaches to the prepared baking dish.

3. In the same bowl, combine almond flour, rolled oats, sliced almonds, melted coconut oil, and ground cinnamon. Mix until crumbly.

4. Sprinkle the almond-oat mixture evenly over the peaches in the baking dish.

5. Bake in the preheated oven for 35-40 minutes, or until the topping is golden brown and the peaches are bubbling.

6. Remove from the oven and let cool slightly before serving.

- Nutritional Info:

  - Calories: 220

  - Carbohydrates: 30g

 - Protein: 5g

  - Fat: 10g

  - Fiber: 6g

6. Watermelon Granita

- Prep Time: 10 minutes

- Freeze Time: 4 hours

- Servings: 6

- Ingredients:

  - 4 cups seedless watermelon cubes

  - 2 tablespoons fresh lime juice

  - Two tablespoons of honey

  - Fresh mint leaves for garnish (optional)

- Instructions:

1. In a blender, combine seedless watermelon cubes, fresh lime juice, and honey or agave syrup.

2. Blend until smooth.

3. Provide a shallow dish, put the mixture in it and place it in the freezer.

4. Every 30 minutes, use a fork to scrape the mixture, breaking up any ice crystals, until the granita is completely frozen and fluffy, about 3-4 hours.

5. To serve, scoop the watermelon granita into serving glasses or bowls.

6. Garnish with fresh mint leaves, if desired, and serve immediately.

- Nutritional Info:

- Calories: 80

- Carbohydrates: 20g

- Protein: 1g

- Fat: 0g

- Fiber: 1g

CHAPTER SIX

14-Day Meal Plan

Day 1:

- Breakfast: Banana Pudding Parfait

- Lunch: Caribbean Mango and Avocado Salad

- Dinner: Cajun Coleslaw with Jamaican Rice and Peas

Day 2:

- Breakfast: Berry Almond Crisp

- Lunch: Southern Collard Greens Salad

- Dinner: Creole Roasted Sweet Potatoes with Southern Style Green Beans

Day 3:

- Breakfast: Chocolate Avocado Mousse

- Lunch: Pineapple Coconut Sorbet

- Dinner: Jamaican Rice and Peas with Southern Style Green Beans

Day 4:

- Breakfast: Peach Cobbler

- Lunch: Caribbean Mango and Avocado Salad

- Dinner: Creole Roasted Sweet Potatoes with Southern Style Green Beans

Day 5:

- Breakfast: Banana Pudding Parfait

- Lunch: Cajun Coleslaw

- Dinner: Jamaican Rice and Peas with Southern Style Green Beans

Day 6:

- Breakfast: Chocolate Avocado Mousse

- Lunch: Berry Almond Crisp

- Dinner: Pineapple Coconut Sorbet

Day 7

- Breakfast: Peach Cobbler

- Lunch: Southern Collard Greens Salad

- Dinner: Creole Roasted Sweet Potatoes with Cajun Coleslaw

Day 8:

- Breakfast: Banana Pudding Parfait

- Lunch: Caribbean Mango and Avocado Salad

- Dinner: Jamaican Rice and Peas with Southern Style Green Beans

Day 9:

- Breakfast: Berry Almond Crisp

- Lunch: Cajun Coleslaw

- Dinner: Pineapple Coconut Sorbet

Day 10:

- Breakfast: Chocolate Avocado Mousse

- Lunch: Southern Collard Greens Salad

- Dinner: Creole Roasted Sweet Potatoes with Caribbean Mango and Avocado Salad

Day 11:

- Breakfast: Peach Cobbler

- Lunch: Berry Almond Crisp

- Dinner: Jamaican Rice and Peas with Southern Style Green Beans

Day 12:

- Breakfast: Banana Pudding Parfait

- Lunch: Cajun Coleslaw

- Dinner: Pineapple Coconut Sorbet

Day 13:

- Breakfast: Chocolate Avocado Mousse

- Lunch: Caribbean Mango and Avocado Salad

- Dinner: Creole Roasted Sweet Potatoes with Southern Style Green Beans

Day 14:

- Breakfast: Peach Cobbler

- Lunch: Berry Almond Crisp

- Dinner: Jamaican Rice and Peas with Cajun Coleslaw

As we come to the end of "Diabetes Cookbook for Black People," we reflect on the journey we've taken together through the rich tapestry of flavors, cultures, and traditions that define Black cuisine. This cookbook has been more than just a collection of recipes; it's been a celebration of heritage, health, and community. Through these pages, we've explored the vibrant colors and bold flavors of Southern comfort food, the exotic spices and tropical fruits of the Caribbean, and the wholesome ingredients and nourishing dishes that sustain us on our journey to better health. We've shown that managing diabetes doesn't mean sacrificing flavor or enjoyment, but rather embracing a diverse and balanced diet that empowers us to live our best lives.

From hearty breakfasts to satisfying main courses and indulgent desserts, each recipe in this book has been carefully crafted to nourish both body and soul. Whether you're cooking for yourself, your family, or your community, these recipes offer a taste of home and a path to wellness.

But our journey doesn't end here. As you continue to explore the joys of cooking and eating, remember that food is more than just sustenance; it's a reflection of who we are and where we come from. By embracing the flavors of our heritage and nourishing our bodies with wholesome ingredients, we honor the traditions of our ancestors while building a healthier future for generations to come.

So let us continue to gather around the table, share stories, and savor the flavors of life. With each meal we prepare and enjoy, let us celebrate the richness of our culture and the gift of good health. Together, we can create a world where diabetes is no longer a barrier, but a bridge to a brighter tomorrow.

Thank you for joining us on this culinary journey. May your plates be filled with love, flavor, and abundance, today and always.

Warm regards,

Diane J. Hays